Bone Broth Boost: An Intensive 7-Day Plan

by

Vanessa S. Castaneda

Table of Contents

Introduction

Step into a world where health trumps passing trends and tradition reigns supreme. Despite the ebb and flow of passing wellness fads, the Bone Broth Diet remains unshakable, exhibiting a time-honored simplicity that has stood the test of time. Within the pages of this intensive 7-day plan, you will begin on a journey to discover the profound and long-term advantages of incorporating bone broth into your daily routine.

Beyond the transitory clamor of quick solutions, this guide invites you to investigate the fundamental nourishment that bone broth provides—nutrition not only for your body but also for your whole well-being. It's more than a diet; it's an invitation to reconnect with our ancestors' knowledge, to draw into the great healing potential of a broth that has seen centuries of health and vibrancy.

As we navigate the complexities of modern wellness, let this guide be your compass, guiding you through a week-long immersion into the transformative potential of the Bone Broth Diet. Embrace the richness of a practice that has sustained generations, and discover how, in just seven days, you can revitalize your body, soothe your soul, and embark on a path towards enduring well-being. Welcome to a journey where simplicity meets profound nourishment—a journey where the tradition of bone broth becomes the cornerstone of your vibrant, modern health story.

Chapter 1: Unlocking the Liquid Gold"

The Ancient Practice of Creating Bone Broth

Bone broth, a nourishing concoction made from bones, marrow, and connective tissues, has its origins in ancient civilizations around the world. This time-honored technique originated out of frugality and necessity, ensuring that no part of an animal was wasted. Bone broth was a foundational dietary staple in many civilizations, valued not just for its fortifying and sustaining capabilities but also for its therapeutic qualities. Ancient healers prescribed it for a variety of diseases, recognizing its healing and rejuvenating properties. Making bone broth is an easy yet meaningful process. To extract the maximum amount of nutrients, such as minerals, collagen, and amino acids, bones are slow-simmered for lengthy hours, frequently with vegetables, herbs, and spices. This methodical heating procedure, which can take up to a day, breaks down the bones and connective tissues, creating a broth that is rich in minerals. Bone broth has long been associated with healing and sustenance, providing warmth and food to people who drink it. The fact that almost all ancient civilizations still included it in their meals attests to its essential importance for human health and culinary tradition.

Nutrient-Rich Composition

Bone broth is well-known for its high nutritional value, making it a health-promoting powerhouse. As it simmers, the bones and connective tissues release a plethora of critical nutrients into the broth, transforming it into a healing potion. The following are the fundamental components that make bone broth a nutritional treasure:

1. **Collagen**: This essential protein, found in bone broth, is the foundation of skin, hair, nails, bones, and joints. Cooking the bones releases collagen into the broth, which, when consumed, can aid with skin

elasticity and joint health and may help reduce the appearance of aging.

2. **Amino Acids:** Bone broth has a high concentration of amino acids, the building blocks of proteins. It includes glycine, proline, and glutamine, among others. Glycine aids the body's detoxification and digesting processes, aids in the creation of glutathione (a powerful antioxidant), and promotes peaceful sleep. Proline improves skin health, but glutamine is essential for gut health and immune function.

3. **Minerals**: The slow simmering process extracts minerals from the bones into the broth, such as calcium, magnesium, phosphorus, silicon, sulfur, and trace minerals. These nutrients are in a readily absorbable form, making bone broth an excellent way to replenish the body's mineral reserves, promoting bone density and overall health.

4. **Gelatin**: As the soup cools, it may gel, indicating that it contains gelatin. Gelatin, generated from collagen, has gut-healing

characteristics and can help maintain healthy bones, promote joint health, and aid digestion. It serves as a protein sparer, allowing the body to make better use of the proteins in the diet.

Chapter 2: 7-Day Journey to Vitality"

7-day Guideline Outlining when to Include Bone Broth in Meals.

Embark on a 7-day journey of transformation by adding bone broth to your daily meals. This step-by-step approach will guide you through a week of consuming bone broth to enhance your intestinal health, improve joint function, and provide a nutrient-rich boost to your overall well-being.

Day 1: Introducing Bone Broth

- **Breakfast**: Start the day with a warm cup of bone broth. Its calming characteristics gradually wake up the digestive system while also providing hydration.
- **Lunch**: Make a mild vegetable soup using bone broth as the foundation. This familiar dish introduces your body to the benefits of bone broth.

- **Dinner**: Cook rice or quinoa in bone broth to improve the nutrition of your meal.

Day 2: Gut Health Focus

- **Breakfast**: Start with bone broth and add a pinch of sea salt for electrolytes. A small cup of bone broth can satisfy hunger while also providing gut-healing amino acids.
- **Lunch**: A salad with a bone broth-based vinaigrette is a refreshing way to incorporate its benefits.
- **Dinner**: Make a bone broth-based stew or casserole with lean meats and vegetables as the main elements.

Day 3: Joint Support

- **Breakfast**: Bone broth with a pinch of turmeric, known for its anti-inflammatory effects, promotes joint health.
- **Lunch**: A bone broth soup with leafy greens and beans contains protein and antioxidants.

- **Dinner**: Serve bone broth gravy with your dinner as a delightful way to incorporate it into your diet.

Day 4: Midweek Boost

- **Breakfast**: Begin with a bone broth smoothie, blended with fruits and vegetables for a nutritious start.
- **Lunch**: A bone broth-based Asian noodle soup can be both refreshing and satisfying.
- **Dinner**: Steam veggies in bone broth to enhance flavor and nutrition.

Day 5: Nutrition for Skin and Hair

- **Breakfast**: A mug of bone broth with a squeeze of lemon to promote skin health.
- **Lunch**: Quinoa salad infused with bone broth and topped with nuts and seeds for extra fats that nourish the skin.
- **Dinner**: Make a fish meal with bone broth that is high in omega-3 fatty acids for healthy skin and hair.

Day 6: Immune Boost

- **Breakfast**: Bone broth with ginger and garlic helps boost the immune system.
- **Lunch**: A spicy bone broth soup with vegetables to energize and replenish nutrients.
- **Dinner**: Chicken soup made with bone broth, which is proven to enhance the immune system.

Day 7: A Full Circle

- **Breakfast**: Begin with your now-familiar cup of warm bone broth to reflect on the week's progress.
- **Lunch**: To celebrate the end of the week, make a delicious bone broth stew with your favorite veggies and proteins.
- **Dinner**: End the week with a simple, comfortable bone broth sip before bed, laying the groundwork for continued wellness.

Potential Benefits:

Bone broth is known for its high collagen content, which can help reinforce and repair the lining of the digestive tract. This can result in improved gut health, better digestion, reduced inflammation, and fewer symptoms of gut-related disorders like IBS (irritable bowel syndrome) or leaky gut syndrome. Bone broth also contains natural substances like glucosamine and chondroitin sulfate, which can benefit joint health. Regular consumption of bone broth can help reduce joint pain and inflammation, making it a crucial dietary supplement for people with arthritis or other joint problems. Another significant benefit of bone broth is its high concentration of essential minerals, including calcium, magnesium, phosphorus, and trace minerals. This makes bone broth a nutrient-dense boost for overall health.

Chapter 3: Flavors Beyond Tradition"

Inventive Method to Enhance the Flavor of Bone Broth with Veggies, Herbs, and Spices.

Exploring the realm of bone broth does not require you to stick to conventional recipes. This chapter will help you enhance the flavor profile of your bone broth and enjoy every drink by experimenting with different herbs, spices, and vegetables. Here are some inventive methods to add colorful flavors and textures to your broth, along with some basic recipes and combos to get you started.

Herb Infusion

Herbs add a refreshing and aromatic depth to bone broth. For a refreshing twist, try the following combinations:

- **Parsley and Bay Leaves**: Incorporate parsley stems and bay leaves in the final hour of boiling to provide a delicate, earthy flavor.
- **Rosemary and Thyme**: Add a sprig of rosemary and a few thyme branches during the last 30 minutes of simmering your broth for a Mediterranean flair.

Spice It Up

Spices may elevate your bone broth from ordinary to exceptional. Consider the following additions:

- **Turmeric and Black Pepper**: Incorporate a teaspoon of turmeric and a few cracks of black pepper to brighten the color and give anti-inflammatory benefits.
- **Ginger and Garlic**: Simmer ginger slices and garlic cloves to make a warming, immune-boosting soup.

Vegetable Varieties

Vegetables not only provide additional nutrients to the soup, but they also offer depth of flavor. Experiment with:

- **Mushrooms**: Add sliced shiitake mushrooms for umami-packed soup.
- **Fennel**: Chunks of fennel can add a subtle anise-like flavor, making them ideal for people looking for a unique taste profile.

Easy Recipes and Taste Combinations

- **Lemongrass and Coconut Broth**: For an Asian twist, add lemongrass stalks, a can of coconut milk, and a splash of fish sauce to your broth. Garnish with rice noodles and fresh cilantro.
- **Spicy Tomato Broth**: Combine tomato paste, chili flakes, and smoked paprika for a flavorful base for soups and stews.
- **Golden Bone Broth**: Add turmeric, ginger, and lemon juice for a visually appealing and health-boosting broth.

Improving Your Bone Broth

- **Roasting Bones**: Before simmering, roast your bones in the oven until browned. This procedure enhances the flavor and color of the broth.
- **Acidic Touch**: Adding a dash of apple cider vinegar might help extract more minerals from the bones. It also imparts a little tanginess to the finished product.
- **Seasonal Touch**: Don't be afraid to use seasonal vegetables and herbs. They deliver fresh flavors while also connecting you to the natural cycle.

By accepting these innovative ideas, you'll discover that bone broth provides an adaptable base for a wide range of culinary excursions. Whether you drink it straight or incorporate it into meals, these additions ensure that your bone broth journey is both healthy and delicious.

Chapter 4: "The Intermittent Twist"

Intermittent Fasting and its Possible Synergies with Bone Broth.

Integrate intermittent fasting into your bone broth journey to fully realize its potential. This chapter explores the connections between intermittent fasting and bone broth, demonstrating how the two practices can work together to maximize their advantages. Discover the simplicity of introducing fasting windows into your daily routine and adopt a holistic approach to health and wellness.

Intermittent Fasting

Intermittent fasting is about generating strategic meal windows rather than limiting one's intake. It permits your body to alternate between feeding and fasting, which promotes metabolic flexibility and the use of stored energy. The beauty is in its simplicity and adaptability to different lifestyles.

Synergies with Bone Broth:

- **Fasting and Autophagy**: Intermittent fasting triggers autophagy, a process in which cells eliminate damaged components. Fasting with bone broth delivers necessary nutrients during the fasting period, which aids in cellular repair and renewal
- **Gut Rest and Healing**: Fasting allows the digestive system to rest, which reduces stress on the gut. Bone broth, with its gut-healing characteristics, serves as a moderate food source during these periods, promoting a healthy gut ecosystem.
- **Satiety and Control**: Bone broth's rich, nutritious composition helps boost feelings of satiety, making it easier to stick to fasting periods. This can help improve portion control during mealtime.

Integrating Fasting Windows:

- **12/12 Method**: Start with a 12-hour fasting window overnight, then gradually increase it to 14 or 16 hours. Break your fast with a cup of bone broth, which provides a gentle introduction to nutrition.
- **Alternate-Day Fasting**: Set aside particular days for intermittent fasting and consume bone broth during the fasting time. On non-fasting days, eat balanced meals with bone broth.
- **Time-Restricted Eating**: Set a daily eating window that includes enough time for fasting. Begin with a warm cup of bone broth, which will fuel you throughout the day.

Practical Tips for Success:

- **Stay Hydrated**: Hydration is essential during fasting periods. In addition to bone broth, drink water, herbal teas, and electrolyte-rich drinks.

- **Listen to Your Body**: Pay attention to hunger and fullness signals. Bone broth can be a grounding and gratifying factor when fasting, but it's important to consider individual needs.
- **Gradual Progression**: If you're new to intermittent fasting, begin with shorter fasting windows and gradually increase them as your body adjusts.

Embracing holistic wellness.

When paired with the nutritional assistance of bone broth, intermittent fasting transforms into a comprehensive approach to wellness. Beyond weight loss, it provides opportunities for cellular repair, improved energy utilization, and a healthy relationship with food. This chapter urges you to investigate the powerful synergy between fasting and bone broth, which will pave the road for a healthier and more vibrant life.

Chapter 5: On-the-Go Nutrition

Ways to Incorporate Bone Broth into Hectic Lifestyles, such as Portable Choices or Quick Meals.

Maintaining a balanced diet in today's fast-paced world can be challenging. However, this chapter reveals the secrets to smoothly incorporating bone broth into your on-the-go lifestyle. Explore practical methods, portable solutions, and quick recipes that will allow you to reap the nutritional benefits of bone broth, no matter how hectic your schedule becomes.

Portable Options

- **Bone Broth in a Thermos**: Purchase a high-quality thermos to keep your bone broth warm for several hours. It's a simple, spill-proof way to transport the soothing elixir wherever your day takes you.

- **Single-Serve Packets**: Select single-serve, powdered bone broth packets. Simply mix it with boiling water to create a simple cup of bone broth that does not require refrigeration.
- **Pre-packaged Bone Broth**: Many supermarkets now sell shelf-stable bone broth. These are small enough to fit in your backpack or work drawer, making them a convenient alternative.

Simple and Fast Recipes

- **Bone Broth Smoothie**: For a hydrating and nutrient-rich smoothie that you can drink on the go, blend bone broth with your preferred fruits, veggies, and a small amount of ice.
- **Instant Noodle Upgrade**: Use bone broth instead of the spice packet for healthier and tastier instant noodles.
- **Microwave-cup Soups**: Keep a cup and a container of bone broth at your desk. Mix with leftover proteins, grains, or

vegetables to make a fast microwave mug soup.

Common Challenges and Solutions.

- **Time constraints**: Prepare bone broth in batches over the weekend and freeze it in ice cube trays. Add a few cubes to boiling water for a quick cup whenever you need it.
- **Limited Kitchen Access**: For limited kitchen access, opt for portable options such as single-serve packets or shelf-stable pre-packaged bone broth.
- **Taste Fatigue**: To avoid taste fatigue, experiment with different flavor combinations, such as herbs, spices, or lemon juice, to keep things interesting.

Maintaining Consistency

- **Schedule Bone Broth Breaks**: Set aside certain periods in your schedule for bone broth breaks, such as mid-morning, afternoon, or evening. Consistency is essential.

- **Set up a Bone Broth Station**: Store bone broth at work or in your car for quick pick-me-ups.
- **Incorporate Existing Habits**: Combine bone broth consumption with current routines, such as commuting, to ensure that it becomes a part of your daily routine.

Nourishing Moments of Motion

By overcoming the challenges of a hectic existence with practical solutions, this chapter enables you to reap the nourishing advantages of bone broth wherever you go. Whether it's a sip from a thermos during a meeting or a quick bone broth smoothie on your commute, this on-the-go nutrition advice can keep your wellness journey on track.

Chapter 6: "Results and Reflection"

As you near the end of your 7-day bone broth trip, it's important to consider the possible consequences and changes that may have occurred. This chapter provides a roadmap to understanding the transforming impacts of introducing bone broth into your routine and invites self-reflection on how this easy addition fits into your health path.

Possible Outcomes in Seven-Day

- **Gut Harmony**: Improved digestion and possible relief from digestive discomforts broth's nutritious qualities promote gut health.
- **Joint Comfort**: Improved joint support, with the collagen, glucosamine, and chondroitin in bone broth supporting joint health.
- **Vibrant Energy**: A nutrient-dense surge that promotes improved vigor and persistent energy all day.

- **Skin Glow**: Bone broth contains collagen and amino acids, which may contribute to skin elasticity and glow.
- **Balanced Wellness**: Bone broth and intermittent fasting together support immune system function, cellular repair, and metabolic flexibility, resulting in a sense of overall well-being.

Assisted Self-Examination

- **Journal Your Experience**: Keep track of your emotions, vitality, and any discernible adjustments to your digestion, joint comfort, or skin condition. This gives you a physical copy of your travel journal.
- **Listen to Your Body**: Observe your body's reaction when you add the bone broth. Do you feel particularly balanced or invigorated in any areas?
- **Connect with Your Wellness Objectives**: Consider how consuming bone broth will help you achieve your overall health objectives. Does it fit in with the lifestyle

you want to lead and improve your general well-being?

- **Celebrate Small Victories**: Recognize any beneficial developments, no matter how minor. Celebrate the decision you've seized for your health.

Moving Forward

- **Continued Integration**: Consider making bone broth a regular part of your routine. Discover your rhythm, whether it's a morning cup, a soup base, or a mid-afternoon sip.
- **Adaptation and Exploration**: Recognise that each individual's journey is unique. If you have difficulties, look into adjustments or new flavor combinations that suit your tastes.
- **Share Your Experience**: If you see positive results, consider sharing your story with friends or online communities. Your observations may encourage others to go on their bone broth quest.

Beyond 7 Days

While seven days may provide a snapshot of the possible advantages of bone broth, this chapter urges you to see it as the start of a long-term journey toward holistic health. By reflecting on your experiences and connecting them to your health objectives, you establish the groundwork for ongoing progress and well-being beyond the first week. Accept the journey, appreciate your accomplishments, and remember that every small step leads to a healthier, more vibrant you.

Conclusion

In conclusion, this 7-day adventure through the Bone Broth Diet has been more than just a culinary experiment; it has demonstrated the enduring strength of good customs. Consider the progress you've made towards holistic well-being over the last week—perhaps improved digestion, increased energy, or a renewed appreciation for bone broth, an ancient elixir.

This program is more than just a temporary routine; it's a catalyst for long-term improvement. Allow the things you've gained on this journey to become ingrained in your daily life as you move forward. Whether you continue to enjoy a daily cup of bone broth, experiment with new flavor combinations, or share your experiences with others, know that you've set the foundation for long-term vitality. Simplicity is frequently the key to the complex puzzle of health. You've had a sneak peek at the transformative power of mindful eating and how it may enhance your general well-being with the help of the ageless wisdom of the bone broth diet. I hope that the balance of history and contemporary medicine will steer your path going forward so that the advantages of this 7-day jumpstart last and improve your health for days on end.